HEALTH IS WEALTH

OWN YOURS!

CAREY ROSS

Published by Spines
ISBN: 979-8-89383-217-4

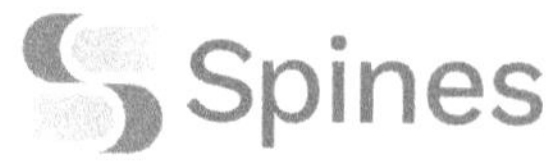

A practical guide to owning and achieving
Total Optimal Health

How I went from a BMI of 32.5 to 22.5 and maintained optimal health for Life! 16 years and counting.

CONTENTS

DEDICATION

I would like to dedicate this book to my beloved and deceased mother Virginia Jean Ross and my deceased father Rudolph Ramsey Ross, who both taught me hard work, dedication, sacrifice and to believe in myself. As one of their children, I am grateful for the example in the time-tested principles of perseverance demonstrated in their lives. Although they are no longer with me their spirits influence me daily to pursue the best life and to believe in myself and others while seeking the better good and to share knowledge and resources with others expecting nothing in return. It is in that spirit that I saw them live out their lives and that I write this book and dedicate this writing to all those who would read it and apply its principles mentioned that they may achieve optimal health through natural means consistent with the longevity of health and wealth to the full and until it overflows.

ACKNOWLEDGMENT

I give honor to my creator God and the power of His Son and Spirit who lives within me for without Him I am nothing.

To my children who are the joys of my life and who have stood by my side and made life truly an inspiration.

To my grandchildren, and future leaders of our world, I am so grateful and I truly feel rich to be a father and grandfather to my amazing family.

I also am grateful to my many healthcare colleagues, role models, mentors in business, and spiritual leaders all of whom collectively have influenced me to serve my community with excellence. I also acknowledge the amazing vegan chef who has helped me navigate the plant-based community with love and support. I will always be grateful for our time together!

I lastly wish to acknowledge my ancestors and all those who lived before me and have contributed to my life for without them also, I would not be.

INTRODUCTION

I watched my grandfather die as a child. My healthcare journey of over thirty-five years in the healthcare industry began sitting by my grandfather's hospital bed watching him slowly die of prostate cancer. I was a little boy close to 10 years old. The hospital room experience changed my life forever as I saw my six-foot-five-inch hero dwindle to mere skin and bones within weeks right before my young eyes.

How did this happen and what could be done in the future to avoid this untimely painful death? My grandfather was a tall physically fit handsome man. He was always well dressed for business and he possessed the finer things in life, so I thought!

I can remember the fishing trips on his private boat that were so much fun. My brothers and I would get so excited when it became time to go see Grandad and little did we know he had been given a short time to live due to a diagnosis of cancer.

He lived a prosperous life and owned multiple

properties in an era when money was tight and opportunities to prosper were few and hard to come by. My grandfather taught me the value of owning real estate and the finer things in life when my immediate surroundings displayed poverty, unhealthy eating choices, and many sick and overweight individuals who seemed to be comfortable living in such dire environments.

In contrast to his life my immediate surroundings included very few supermarkets, many fast-food restaurants, and liquor stores abounded in my immediate community. It appeared as if we lived in different worlds while residing in the same city limits. His life in my view as a child was so good that I found it hard to believe he was dying at the young age of sixty-nine. He suffered through an extended hospital stay that included intense medical treatment and chemotherapy along with many needle sticks withdrawing blood samples for testing. As the treatment proceeded his appetite diminished as it became too difficult to keep solid food in his stomach. The hospital began feeding him through a tube in the last few days of his life. Ultimately my hero would die as I sat next to his bed for days hoping and expecting him to get back to those immaculate living conditions I longed to experience and my personal favorite was his very cool fishing boat!

My wished recovery for him never happened and as I sat next to his bed until the final hours and eventual minutes and final seconds there would be no recovery and the process of burial began while in the same room hoping he would come home! The experience left me in shock, sad, and angry that I had lost the one person who I looked up to and he was my grandad.

1

MY FIRST HEALTH CRISIS

In January 2013 I became intimately aware of just how important your health is. For years I observed my weight fluctuate depending on the pressures of life. I recall working 60-90 hours per week and stuffing my mouth with any warm foods that I could easily access and were satisfying to my taste. Salt and sugar were the dominant taste desires. Eating in such a careless way led to my weight reaching a whopping two-hundred and seventy-plus pounds. As I stood six feet five inches I could barely walk upstairs without losing my breath! Playing in the backyard with my youngest son a family member snapped a picture of me leaning over to pick up a basketball with no shirt on. The picture told a story of just how bad my health had become. My mid-section was close to 44-46 inches wide. My physique was non-existent, and I was shocked to see how far off my ideal body weight I had become. In a mad rush to overturn that bad picture of myself that I could not get out of my mind, I sought the services of a personal trainer. I even went through several at-home fitness programs and achieved substantial weight loss. However, the short-term gains seem to come back as I didn't change my eating habits to match my desire for better health.

After months of up and down results I committed on a cold January morning to working out with a dedicated personal trainer. I planned to participate in my first Iron Man event to keep myself on track to sustained weight loss and better overall health. Recall that picture of my disgusting figure while picking up that basketball in my backyard while playing with my son?

I was preparing physically for a marathon that I would never participate in. My personal trainer and I began the long journey of getting my body in the best physical shape that I can imagine. This included many calisthenics, weightlifting, eating right, and rest. This included drinking large amounts of water and taking supplements to keep my body going and I believed I was on my way to what I like to call the "Ironman physique".

My trainer and I fully engaged as he was showing me all of the techniques to build muscle he was testing my mental fortitude and was driving me for what I had in my mind as the perfect physique. On one particular day, I was doing squats with extra weights and I'll never forget it felt so good to continue to push heavier weights. In fact, I was intrigued just how far I could challenge my body and I was eager to see massive change. This all came to a screeching halt when I went down on my right knee trying to push too much weight for that conditioning exercise.

I went down abruptly on one knee thinking nothing of it and soon realized I needed to lessen the amount of free weight that I was lifting. It was a little embarrassing to me that I had not properly balanced the approach with the amount of weight for the lift. After going down on one knee with extra weight on my shoulders and in my hands I thought nothing of hitting my right knee hard on the rubber mat. Within days of this incident, I noticed my breathing started to change. I began sweating profusely at night and had difficulty breathing with just normal activities. Being the hard worker that I am I did not pay total attention to my body and kept up the very demanding routine of a 60 to 70 plus hours work week driving for 3 ½ to 4 hours a day during my daily commute.

All while getting about 4 to 6 ½ hours' sleep and this led to a complete breakdown of my total health. As I remember it started slow with sweating clammy skin difficulty breathing and of course I began to seek medical attention as my symptoms worsened. These worsening symptoms included skin color changes inability to sleep throughout the night even though it was limited to 4 to 6 hours and I began to spit up what I now know were blood clots that had formed in my lungs.

I engaged the healthcare system and was initially diagnosed with pneumonia. This included a regimen of medications and advice to limit my activity and get more rest. I recall the many prescriptions that I was offered to sleep at night and on the surface it seemed like the right thing to do. I was offered codeine cough syrup and something inside me said this is not pneumonia. As a result, I did not take the medication and I returned to see my physician to complain that my symptoms were worsening.

This all transpired within days which turned into weeks

which turned into months. One day while working with what I now know were blood clots in my lungs my corporate manager noticed that my physical appearance had changed. She said to me you don't look okay can you go to the ER and get checked out. I stated that I had done so and I was under the care of my physician while trying to work. She noticed that I was physically sweating and my energy levels were much different than she was accustomed to. She insisted that I go see a physician right away!

Upon visiting the doctor at the direction of my manager I learned after weeks and months of trial and error that my body had produced blood clots in my lungs and I was in grave danger. I recall finally seeing a pulmonologist who had gone through many different evaluations to determine why I was not getting better and on this particular visit, he offered a new regimen of antibiotics because again he thought it was pneumonia and he gave me a list of medications to take to the pharmacy.

While sitting in the pharmacy waiting room to obtain the medication my name was called by the receptionist at the pharmacy counter. I remember walking up barely able to move to the counter to say I was here and was told by the receptionist that my pulmonologist was looking for me and to return to his office immediately.

As soon as I finished that interaction my pulmonologist was walking toward the pharmacy to reconnect with me as my chest X-ray had shown and confirmed that there were clots forming in my lungs and I needed a different course of medical treatment as soon as possible.

I walked back to my pulmonologist's office, and he sat me down and said I need you to listen very closely. You are in very grave danger and your chest X-ray shows that you have multiple blood clots that have formed in your lungs. I need you to return to the emergency room to be treated with thrombolytic medication otherwise known as blood clot-busting medication immediately. Of course, this was not the news that I was expecting as I was still functioning albeit with extra effort. I did not feel that I was in danger. So I began negotiating with my physician about the time I needed to get more work done and see my family rather than take care of myself.

My physician exercised extreme patience slowed down and showed me the X-rays that demonstrated multiple blood clots were forming in my lungs and that I needed a different course of treatment immediately. My doctor arranged for me to go to the emergency room closer to my family home which allowed me to drive another 45 minutes East which was not ideal given the situation I found myself in. I remember arriving at my son's school to arrange for a different pickup as I needed to get to the emergency room. This particular day at my son's school was the mother-and-son dance night. As I drove up to the school I could hear the music and the fun festivities which were very exciting. As I exited my vehicle I began running out of energy just to walk from the public street to the entrance to the dance to announce that I was on my way to the emergency room. It took so much effort just to make it halfway and I simply could not go another step.

I had never felt so helpless in all of my life. My life flashed before me on the canvas of my imagination as I could hear my sons enjoying the dance and I was in the battle for my life. As I decided to get back in the car and drive to the emergency room, I was afraid and I began to think will I survive this health crisis if I do not, will anyone know what happened to me?

My breathing was so difficult and my chest was so tight it felt as if someone was stabbing me in my back and my front at the same time! I finally made it after much energy spent in the emergency room and checked myself in for emergent medical care.

The physicians so poised and professional walked into the triage room and stated to me you are in a very dangerous situation. The clots have formed in your lungs and you have lost 1/3 of your capacity in one lung. My doctor began to go over the treatment options which included thrombolytic medication to dissolve the clots and a more conservative heparin approach which took longer to dissolve the clots but was less risky and the third option was to do nothing and immediate death was closer than I'd like to admit. I remember lying on that cold gurney replaying in my mind the three options my physician was sharing with me. At the moment I had never felt so alone, scared, and fragile while also feeling like I was on the edge of life and death.

My physician restated we did not have much time I needed to be admitted to the hospital immediately regardless of which option I chose. I didn't know who to call because I had never faced such a health crisis in my 40-plus years of living. Within minutes my physician came back into the room and he said what are you going to do? He restated my options and reminded me that if I did nothing I risk immediate death and the conservative approach with heparin injections would take time and there was still a danger that I needed to move away from to decrease my risk of premature death.

Out of all of the three options provided to me I chose to be admitted to the hospital for the first time in my life and receive heparin drips over the next few days. The other option of the thrombolytic medication included side effects that I could bleed out and die right in the emergency room. The statements of my physician were like hearing the worst news I have ever heard in my life. As I stated I didn't know who to call I didn't know which option would get me out of danger and allow me to return to a demanding lifestyle. As I settled in for the night at the hospital and began the heparin treatment offered to me I noticed my symptoms began to shift. By the second day of hospitalization, I was able to breathe without pain but I still had a long road ahead and my recovery was just getting underway.

By the third day in the hospital, my physician came in to remind me that I was still in danger as the clots were forming more rapidly than he had initially diagnosed. Again fear began to cloud my judgment as I had never been hospitalized in my life. I recall laying in the hospital bed very cold at night hearing the buzzing of all the machines around me and I thought what am I going to do to get out of this setting this is not where I want to be nor is this where I want to end my life.

After living through the days in the hospital and remembering the pressure mounting as I felt like my life was on pause, I decided I must check out of the hospital to meet a pressing demand in my personal life. I had been recently served divorce papers and I felt I could not miss that upcoming court date. Confused, recovering albeit slowly, and with pressing personal family demands, I chose to leave the care of the hospital setting.

I recall my physician stating to me that if you check out now you put your life in your own hands and this is considered checking out against medical advice! I felt I had no choice but to take the risk to get my personal life in order.

As I prepared for discharge from the hospital I recall receiving doses of heparin to be injected at home into my stomach and being told that I would have to take blood thinners for the rest of my life.

The discharge instructions also included staying away from things that I love like green leafy delicious kale not being able to play contact sports and being told that I could never ride a motorcycle again as all these things could cause trauma which could create new blood clots that could flow up to my brain and potentially cause stroke or flow to my heart which could lead to cardiac arrest and even immediate death!

As I waited and listened to all of these options of post-discharge care that I would have to administer to myself, I thought wow how did I get here? What was going on in my life that I thought physical fitness was so important that I would ignore my health in a way that I didn't intend to do but I found myself having to daily intake heparin and make drastic lifestyle changes that I never thought were even a remote possibility for someone like me.

Of course, this is a process that allows one to self-reflect and examine lifestyle and many other contributing factors that landed me in that poor state of health. My discharge diagnosis included pulmonary embolism and loss of 1/3 of my right lung capacity. These are very serious health issues and I was quite frankly overwhelmed by how fast this all happened.

As I treated myself with heparin injections in the home setting I began to experience depression, loss of concentration, limited ability to even talk for extended periods and I was afraid to fall asleep. I recall learning of several members of my community who had recently experienced pulmonary embolism and two people I knew of had died in their sleep from the medications that were prescribed to help them sleep.

These were trying times that I had never experienced. I felt lost, alone, depressed, afraid, and angry all directed inward as I inwardly blamed myself for all that was happening. I had days of deep depression thinking about what would happen to my children if I didn't show up to divorce court. Who would take care of them and did I work to achieve enough resources to support them if I didn't live through this health crisis? What would my siblings think? Who would tell them in detail what had happened to me? I thought about my mother's untimely death at age forty-seven. Is it my time to die and the days and weeks ahead seemed so difficult to ponder?

As I attempted to sleep at night, the thoughts seemed to flood my mind intensely and I wanted to take the medication as the pain to breathe at night was unbearable. Somehow, I made it through with the assistance of my family and friends. I had never needed anyone to take care of me during a health crisis and I learned just who and what real friends and family are made of.

2

HEALTHCARE IN THE UNITED STATES

THE HEALTH INDUSTRY in the United States has made amazing technological advances in cardiac care, pulmonary medicine, cancer care treatment, screening tools, radiology diagnostics, laboratory medicine, and pharmacological advances, acute care along with amazing healthcare teams and dedicated physicians, nurses, and ancillary staff all aiming to deliver exceptionally high-quality healthcare.

The healthcare teams extend to even the home settings as some family and friends are identified and become qualified caregivers. On many occasions, the teams all work together on behalf of patients who need assistance to gain full health for various reasons. For some patients, the road to full recovery is long, difficult, and sometimes out of reach. For other patients who need minor surgery or routine procedures performed in the outpatient setting, great outcomes can be the norm.

For others in the United States Healthcare setting depending on factors such as geography, age, sex, socioeconomic status, and ethnicity, some of these segments of the US population do not receive optimal care. Care can also be fragmented by fee-for-service health systems and, by that, I mean many handoffs to specialists for things like specialty care, cancer treatment, or even eye care that can lead to mistakes and often bad outcomes for the patients receiving care.

For the most part, close coordination of care is achieved within integrated health systems. For some patients in the fee-for-service health systems, lack of close care coordination can lead to negative outcomes up to and including accidental deaths. If there are no electronic medical records, providers are often unaware of the full medical histories of patients they are treating.

Accidents in US hospitals occur more frequently than we would like to think or admit. One accidental death to the patient's family is one too many and should be avoided at all costs. I as a family member have been on the wrong side of negative healthcare outcomes which might have been prevented if closer care coordination and stronger outpatient prevention programs without bias or racism within them had been offered or delivered.

Far too many times I have lost loved ones to fragmented fee-for-service care delivery systems with uncaring providers and overwhelmed systems of care which has devastated my family and the communities we collectively make up.

I can recall on several occasions untimely deaths of family and friends growing up who went in for routine care like childbirths and some did not make it home alive.

For instance, the Tuskegee Study of Untreated Syphilis

in the Negro Male was a study conducted between 1932 and 1972 by the United States Public Health Service and the Centers for Disease Control and Prevention on a group of nearly 400 African American men with syphilis. The study did not collect informed consent from participants and they did not offer treatment even after it was widely available. The study which is a part of US Healthcare history makes trust in the system difficult for those impacted by the study. These horrible stories have an effect even in the modern times we live in today.

Even though the United States Healthcare Industry has made significant improvements in technology, screening for cancers, drug advances, and more ethnically diverse providers trust is still fragile in some subpopulations.

Some groups even have a mistrust of simple annual physicals which when done regularly can detect and help prevent the progression of serious disease and untimely death.

Furthermore, of all countries in 2020, the United States possessed the highest infant mortality rate at 5.4 deaths per 1000 lives, which is markedly higher than the 1.6 deaths per 1000 lives in Norway, which has the lowest mortality rate. Non-Hispanic blacks infant mortality rates in 2021 were 10.6 compared to non-Hispanic Asians at 3.7.

These important mortality rates by race tell a story of gaps in care that can be fatal for some groups and we as an industrialized nation with one of the most expensive most advanced healthcare systems in the world should and must do better.

3

THE HEALTH INDUSTRY QUICK FIX SOLUTIONS

In the United States, we spend way too much money on quick-fix diet pills and other over-the-counter remedies *that simply do not work!* Some estimates include annual spending in the billions on diet pills alone in the United States. When you throw in supplements and magic potions the annual money spent is way more. Yet despite this annual spending spree we still see alarming rates of obesity, type 1 and type 2 diabetes along with other risk factors which can lead to premature death and chronic disease.

Why do we fall for such schemes? Why do we as a society look for the easy way out instead of working to change deep-seated poor dietary habits and unhealthy relationships with food? Why do we buy the idea that the expensive pill or fake remedy will do what we cannot or are unwilling to do? Could it be pre-programming by well-designed marketing campaigns and ads that make us collectively believe that all we need is a pill instead of a balanced eating routine with built-in daily exercise?

Let us examine our core beliefs and behaviors that make us susceptible to easy, quickly do-it-in-instant items which range from diet pills to get-rich-quick schemes. As one thinks deeply about the ideas of avoiding hard work and slow steady progressive changes to optimal health which when understood and carefully followed can lead to sustained change in behavior which roots the destructive thinking and bad behavior which collectively produce bad results. If we are willing and decide on the following tried and true time-tested methods to achieve optimal health we can change results in favor of healthier living and increased healthy food choices which can prolong life with vitality and strength as a by-product of this proposed changed thinking and opposite approach to the quick fix do it in instant programming many Americans seem to be so stuck in using.

Of course, this is not easy. We do not mean to sound naïve here. To approach this topic of uprooting deep core beliefs associated with food choices and lifestyle some may find it too difficult to even try. The path may seem too daunting and I would offer the scenario of rethinking this short-term pain. Imagine you have worked hard all of your life to achieve something meaningful like a financial portfolio with significant assets. All of a sudden with no warning those progressively built over time assets are seized or stolen to never be enjoyed as planned. Think of the feelings of extreme loss, shock and anger! Think of all the what ifs, did I invest correctly, did I miss red flags etc.

I am suggesting that if we build our lives on quick fix solutions without the hard work of progressive benefits and slow little by little gains and results, we could be gambling with our most precious asset-life! If you think I am being over dramatic research the accidental deaths from global plastic surgery and you will find this is a real problem that can be solved by thinking and taking action consistent with steady tried and true approaches to natural weight loss and ideal body weight goal setting with proper balanced nutrition aligned to support healthy long prosperous living.

That is what owning your health is all about. When you take the time to think, analyze, and uproot bad core beliefs associated with bad eating patterns and a sedentary lifestyle this is owning your health. Think about that nice car or beautiful home or whatever you find in life worth owning and taking care of. Your life is worth much more than anything material, right? So why not abandon the quick fixes and get on the road to better health by doing your research and creating a plan of action suited to your personal health goals? Consult with your healthcare professionals who align with your values of healthy well-balanced living. Get your family and friends involved in your life change strategy. The results can be amazing. I achieved an over 10-point BMI reduction and reached and maintained my ideal body weight with no diet pills or quick-fix solutions. You can too. Why wait? Get started today!

4

MAN MADE DRUGS, THE UNINTENDED HEALTH CONSEQUENCES

No MATTER where you are in the United States or the world on the benefits of man-made synthetic pain-killing drugs the opioid crisis is a perfect example of man-made drugs that have produced unintended consequences of overdose deaths never before observed at least in my lifetime.

For many people the need for pain medicine is real. If you have ever had chronic pain or a need to have surgery the post-operative pain associated with that procedure can be unbearable without some man-made drug assistance. I get that and by no means am I suggesting that all man-made drugs are bad for all and must be avoided. However, when you casually observe the opioid crisis alone in the United States the overdose deaths are alarming and steadily rising with no end in sight.

These are preventable deaths with tragic stories of untimely death that leave families in deep pain, shock, anger, and uphill battles in search of relief due to the deaths of loved ones addicted to painkillers or opioid drugs. The opioid settlements from overdose deaths from overprescribing of these drugs are massive pay-outs of billions of US dollars. However, these payout offers from opioid manufacturers, distributors, and pharmacies to settle various lawsuits against drug companies across the United States will not adequately compensate for loss of life and pain & suffering many families have felt due to these tragic events. The last figure I recall was close to 5 billion US dollars to settle opioid abatements nationwide! Of course, no amount of money will ever be enough to replace a loss of human life.

Now I am all for some type of compensation for those responsible for pushing these death pills on unsuspecting victims who were in search of pain relief legitimate to a cause related to pain from some event and no relief achieved through more conservative approaches could be obtained.

Owning one's health suggested in this writing includes approaches to pain control using natural means including meditation, relaxed breathing, and other homeopathic methods free from man-made synthetic drugs. Additional natural pain relief suggestions include using turmeric, ginger, acupuncture, and Boswellia. In addition, there are many over-the-counter herbs and other proven remedies for natural pain relief. Do your research and consult with your healthcare provider before you accept the quick fix man-made easy solution. The unintended consequences could cost you or your loved ones' lives!

5

THERE MUST BE A BETTER WAY TO LIVE HEALTHY

My plant-based eating journey began with uprooting a deep core belief that food was comfort and that if I had an exceptional meal I should be taking a long nap shortly thereafter consuming such meal. You see I grew up in the Southern United States and my family had access to multiple farms where we grew some of our food and raised cattle such as cows, chickens, pigs, fishing ponds, and such and we also grew many different vegetables all for enjoyable food consumption. In those days you knew the cattle feed and grain you supplied to the farm animals including the fish in our ponds and you pretty much controlled what that looked like and the amounts of additive ingredients and supplements to make the animals grow and the food taste good.

For the most part, we used all-natural ingredients with no harmful chemicals and we processed the food all within the control of the family farm. We had very little outside input and very few if any pesticides added to the vegetables.

In hindsight, most of the vegetables were organic before the term took on modern terms that we look for in supermarkets today to guide us on what is included and not, in that nice red strawberry or dark green avocado!

Growing up as a child, I recall the beautiful Sunday dinners with the menu spread including many favorites including deep southern fried chicken, catfish, t-bone and ribeye steaks, collard greens, yams, macaroni and cheese, green beans, mashed potatoes, cornbread gravy and of course the desserts. The aftermath of post-meal desserts included peach and apple cobbler, sweet potato pie, German chocolate cake, lemon meringue pie, apple pie, seven-up pound cake, bread pudding, and rice pudding just to name a few. I am getting hungry and sleepy just thinking about those fantastic meals from my childhood.

Of course, lots of love and family gatherings went with this homemade food and it made life enjoyable... at least so I thought. I mean, the family gathering part was always a joy but looking back the extra calories from those beautiful food spreads had too much sugar and salt contained in them and I believe these excessive ingredients contributed to many chronic conditions like diabetes, hypertension, and heart disease which took the lives of many of my family members while they were young! To this day, I often wonder if my mother who died at age 47 of a massive heart attack could be alive if she had been on a plant-based eating lifestyle versus the animal-rich high salt and sugar cuisine in the South, also known as soul food. Not to mention the countless aunts and uncles, grandparents and friends who all died way too early in large part in my opinion, from the collective harmful cumulative effects of a bad diet and little to no exercise.

What I have experienced in my 16-plus years of moderate exercise and 10 plus years eating plant-based is that after consuming a meal I feel energized and fueled up for my fast-paced lifestyle. You see part of my uprooting the deep core beliefs about food included deciding to rethink food as fuel for life! I had grown up thinking of food as comfort. I know many people still feel that food is comfort and we even have many comfort food menu items that include, spaghetti Bolognese, smothered chicken, macaroni, and cheese just to name a few. But what is comfort food and where did that title come from?

According to the Cambridge Dictionary comfort food is the type of food that people eat when they are sad or worried, often sweet food or food that people ate as children. I prefer the Cambridge definition of comfort food to make the point that this is the deep-rooted belief about food that I grew up with. That food was almost a drug to soothe pain and enabled one to forget the abject poverty we lived in daily. Growing up with such an unhealthy relationship with food made it very difficult to achieve optimal health. I know the food tastes good but too much of it was not good for us!

As a reflection on my plant-based eating habits, I am delighted to highlight my ideal body weight of 190 US pounds and a BMI of 22.5. That is a ten-point BMI reduction and I have no cravings for salt or sugar. I eat a fun balanced plant-based cuisine that affords me the food as fuel rethinking to run my lifestyle with high energy and mental clarity including glowing skin and no reliance on medications to make it through a day.

For me, the choice to pursue plant-based eating was based on the desire for total health, free from harmful man-made products that can have detrimental effects on my body. Having an understanding of the risk factors from my family history which include: hypertension, diabetes, heart disease, and obesity, I wanted to give myself the best possible chance to succeed with my predetermined health goal. This goal was optimal health drug-free and sustainable for life. This includes daily consumption of organic fruits and vegetables. My morning routine includes first high PH balanced water. Preferably 9-10 PH. Organic strawberries, blueberries, raspberries, and blackberries. I also include organic dates, organic cashews, and organic Goji berries to name a few breakfast daily menu items. I prefer no wrapped food or pre-packaged food as this approach could include harmful items not easily detected by the average person. The more wrapping the more processed food with potentially harmful ingredients.

You may be asking yourself, how expensive is this to maintain? I would say in response that you are worth the initial upfront cost to put organic foods in your body. The projected back-end cost of pricey diets, magic bullet pills that do not work and untimely healthcare costs for medications can more than outweigh the cost of eating the aforementioned items. For dinner, the same approach, whole foods, grains, vegetables, plant-based protein, plant-based cheeses and other tasty plant-based items round out a fully healthy approach that is sustainable over time. As mentioned 16 years and counting and I have not broken the bank exercising and preparing plant-based food items. Not to mention, I am living drug-free with full vitality, energy, and mind clarity which will continue to pay huge dividends as Health is Wealth and I highly suggest you Own Yours!

I will keep modeling the plant-based approach and daily moderate exercise to my family, community, and global community as opportunities present themselves to share how I overcame the risk factors of diabetes, hypertension, and heart failure to achieve optimal health. This is not to say that individuals should throw away or stop taking medications prescribed by licensed physicians. It is my story and my approach to achieving optimal health. Of course, there are other ways to achieve optimal health. Consult with your healthcare professional for the appropriate advice.

There are also many new plant-based restaurants popping up all around my community. Also, some traditional restaurants are now offering plant-based items at reasonable prices to attract plant-based customers. The choice is yours to make and the menu is doable given the explosion of plant-based items in local grocery stores and restaurants. Not to mention the fun of preparing my home-created meals using plant-based items. I could go on. Use your creativity to start a new journey toward optimal health. Try it, what do you have to lose other than some potential unwanted pounds and potential avoidance of risk factors that can turn into diseases no one wants if they could avoid them? It's a fun plant-based journey and I am committed for life!

Do you still think plant-based eating is too good to be true? I know of a cardiologist who transformed his practice into prescribing plant-based meals as medicine. He is enjoying a thriving business and has many testimonials of his patients being transformed off of many expensive medications onto plant-based meals which his practice teaches his patients how to make during daily and weekly meal preparation classes.

According to Dr Baxter Montgomery, his mission is to heal his patients through a plant-based lifestyle.

Dr Montgomery's journey to plant-based nutrition began 17 years ago before it was a thing. Dr Montgomery states: "There were several components. I refer to it more as an evolution. I was a busy cardiologist who started my practice in 1997. In cardiology training, I developed some interest in wellness with some rotations in cardiac rehabilitation. When I opened my practice, I started to get to know my patients from a longitudinal standpoint as they turned into lifelong patients."

If my mother had been treated by Dr Montgomery she maybe still alive. A tragic death that I wish could have been avoided: When I was nineteen years old my mother died of a massive heart attack. I will never forget the helpless feelings as I learned the news of my mothers untimely death at 47!

I recall speaking with my mother daily or weekly as I transitioned to the United States Navy Health Care setting on the West Coast of the United States. My mother was my best friend in life. I would call her to ask meal preparation questions as I attempted to make the delicious meals she prepared for me as a child. On several occasions, I would call to learn her secrets in my attempts to make ground beef-based chili amongst other favorites. What a delicious treat. Not to mention the many animal-based additional menu items including fried chicken, baked chicken, and incredible T-bone steaks when we could afford them. In one attempt to reach my mom for meal preparation advice, by phone while stationed at a West Coast Pacific Fleet Naval command hospital, I will never forget the paramedics answered the phone. I thought this must be a mistake as I had just spoken with my mother a few days ago. It was not, she had experienced a massive heart attack while vacuuming the floor of her nice garden townhouse in Memphis Tennessee. She was scheduled to be picked up on this cold Monday night, by my older sister to drive to choir rehearsal as she and my sister were members of a Memphis-based church choir. My mother could sing! I too was a part of the same church choir growing up as a child!

I thought my mother was a picture of strong health. I never remember her ever being sick. She worked a full-time job and had a side hustle during the summer at the minor league baseball team in the Memphis, Tennessee area.

All of a sudden, she was gone. Without warning my mother just dropped dead at the young age of 47. This event changed my life forever and I believe the event of her untimely death propelled me on a journey to improve my own health. Of course, I was in shock initially to think of my mother no longer on the planet or able to talk in person to visit with or simply hear her voice. All of my dreams to repay her for the hard work and sacrifices she made for me and her children I could no longer plan to repay. I felt lost, angry, and depressed, and as a newly trained United States Navy Hospital staff person, it began to set in that none of my world-class training in healthcare would ever benefit my mother. She was gone, way too soon, and I so miss her every day of my life. None of my children or grandchildren ever got to meet my mother!

The year was 1987 and I was just starting my healthcare

career. My heart throbbed with pain to know she died alone and I was working in an acute care hospital learning the many facets of United States healthcare only to feel helpless that none of my training was ever able to save my mother.

After much soul searching and research I learned her death was cardiac-related and began to consider how I could prevent that outcome in my own life. Also during her untimely death in 1987, I learned my firstborn child was on the way within the same month my mother died. What a year, I was devastated at the loss of my mother and within days of arriving back to the West Coast overjoyed to learn of my new firstborn child. It was a girl. I can recall feeling somewhat guilty that my mother had recently passed and I learned the delightful news that I would now be a father.

6

TRANSFORMATION IN MY PHYSICAL HEALTH

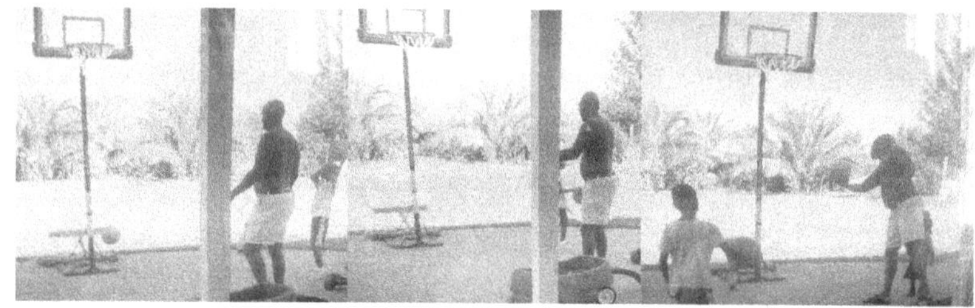

STARTING with a fast from all foods I went from 273 pounds and a Body Mass Index calculation of 32.5 considered obese, to a transformed physique of 190 pounds and a 22.5 BMI with no medications or fad diets!

My journey to optimal health was triggered with that snapped backyard photo while playing with my sons. The picture here on this page captured a moment in time when I was considered obese. As I reviewed the picture and thought of my young sons and their active bright eyes radiating with life, something in me ignited a determined effort to make a real life-sustaining change. This change included research on the best weight loss attempts known to man. I pursued many physical exercise programs and put in the hard work to lose the weight that I had gained.

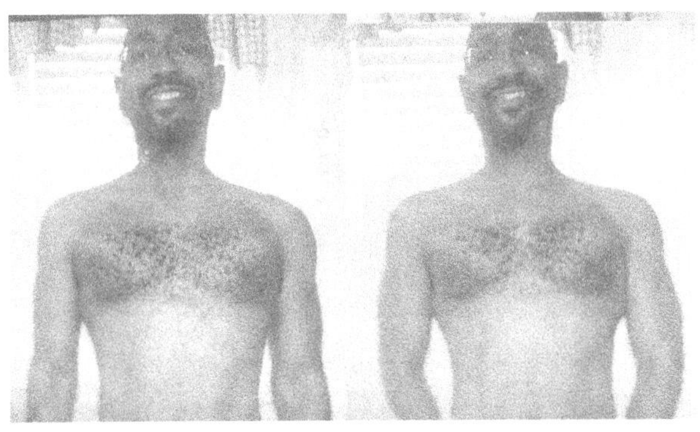

Along with the exercise I began changing my eating habits slowly to more natural plant-based options and I noticed slowly over time the weight loss was being sustained with no overlapping skin sags which thrilled me and inspired me to keep at it! I researched more on plant-based eating combined with exercise and found my new path to sustained life change. That's right, sustained life change! You see, diets and fad diet pills do not work as a long-term solutions to total health. I found that there is no substitute for hard work! If I was to change the bad eating habits I had developed over the years it had to include a decision to change which included regular moderate exercise! As I desired real life-sustaining change I decided to start in my mind by visualizing the new me every day. I found physically fit photos of bodybuilders I admired and I cut out some photos and put them up all around my living spaces.

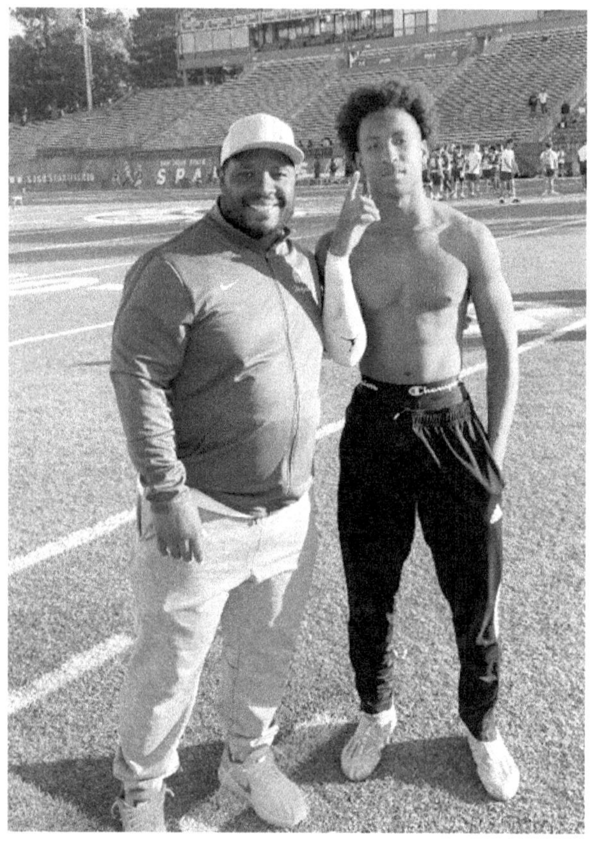

My transformation began as an inside job. There is significant evidence and scientific research that points to the power of imagination and positive thinking aligned with a clear goal. I set my ideal body weight and the new me inside my mind and once that picture was sealed inside it was only a matter of time before it manifested in my physical world. I did it and so can you! It does not matter where you are as long as you decide that you will not stay the same and consider real change. Afterwards there must be a pursuit of education on the health goals you set for yourself. Once you begin educating yourself then I suggest saturation of content relevant to your predetermined goals. For me, I set a target ideal body weight of 190 pounds. I stand 6'5 and a half and decided nothing would stop me from achieving this goal. I am now more than 16 years living my best life and committed to a balanced plant-based eating routine combined with daily moderate exercise up to 5-7 days a week. My son is watching. Pictured during his college football tryouts next to the great Maurice Jones-Drew, my son is pursuing exceptional physical fitness and I'd like to think that I had something to do with that! I also have a son playing college basketball and another playing colleage football. They all are phenomenal athletes in their own right. Not to mention my two grandsons are also athletes. One plays both baseball and basketball and the other grandson plays football. He already has a goal to play in the NFL. He is only 9! Remember: you have an audience watching your daily food choices and that audience includes your family. They are watching, what will you show them? I chose to model health with plant-based eating coupled with daily moderate exercise. The choice is yours to make.

7

HOW TO HELP OTHERS ACHIEVE TOTAL HEALTH BASED ON PERSONAL EXPERIENCE AND RESULTS

OVER THE PAST 16-plus years of moderate daily exercise and 10 plus years of plant-based eating, I have provided insights into better living with a modified lifestyle and a sincere desire to change. I have learned that Genetics may load the gun with built-in physiological characteristics but lifestyle pulls the trigger. By that I mean you may inherit certain genetic risk factors such as hypertension, diabetes, etc, However, one's lifestyle is the key to how these risk factors affect your life. It all starts with how we think about food. Food is fuel for the body to supply needed energy and nourishment for our lifestyle. Not to be confused with eating for comfort, which many overweight individuals routinely do.

"I realized that the most heralded advances of modern medicine are simply mimicking what the healthy body does all by itself. While more people are now living in old age, there is no evidence that the maximum human life span has changed since biblical times, and some of the overall improvement may be due to natural selection, not medical intervention." Payer, L. (1992)

I recall on a cold Christmas Day outside the family home putting up lights standing on the tall ladder with tight-gripped gloves and safety gear to ensure my safety was solid. I had made all the right connections and spaced all the light bulbs just right. Upon safely disembarking from the ladder I made it down to the ground and was delighted to have accomplished the goal of hanging light colored lights all around the house. The next move I made was to lower the tall ladder by clinching both safety release pins on each side of the ladder. I hit the pins too hard and the ladder came down hard and fast with power and landed on my right big toe! Ouch! As the pain routed from my right foot up to my chest and head I recall a huge rush and a release of unaudible sound that came from my mouth. I grabbed my right leg in pain and limped over to the grass thinking I must have crushed my right big toe and would need immediate medical attention to make it through the day. To my surprise as I sat down on the cool green grass and removed my right shoe, not even a bruise was visible even though the pain was intense. As I sat there thinking about why I hit those release pins in error the pain began to subside. The next day as I awakened from sleep I just knew I would see a swollen big toe and redness along with some pain. To my surprise no such bruising or swelling was evident and the pain had been reduced to a mild barely noticeable ache. As I think back clearly there should have been some swelling and even a fracture with the velocity of that drop directly on my right big toe. No such symptoms presented and I never even took a Tylenol for pain day 1 to

2 or any days after. My body seemed to heal on its own with no outside influence.

Your thoughts can lead the way to your ideal state of health. As one famous United Negro College Fund marketing ad indicates: "The mind is a terrible thing to waste".

> "Thoughts become things if you see them in your mind you will hold them in your hand."
>
> BOB PROCTOR

There is a natural order set up in the universe that is in complete balance with all living things. There is a power that thrusts intention into the unseen perils of space and time. This intangible, yet very real force is directing our every move, our every word, our every action, and our every result. This is the power of our thoughts.

We are the magnificent orchestrators of our destiny; we have the power to direct circumstances and get into alignment with the perfect events that could shape everything we want in our lives. This can be repeated to you constantly, but unless you believe it, and reinforce it from within more than you deflect it, you will never know its truth.

As rational people, we constantly downplay the magnitude that we may influence any single aspect of our lives simply by redirecting the route that our thinking has taken us. If you are on a ship that is heading for a big iceberg, you don't just keep pushing forward. You are going to notice on the ships radar something underwater that must be avoided and hopefully grip the edge of the wheel and pull that ship in the opposite direction. Life is the same, yet so many people see the iceberg coming and they continue in the same direction until it's too late.

The majority of the thoughts we think are not our own. We are bombarded through our lives with others enforcing their opinions, judgments, insecurities, and prejudices that we barely have enough time to form our own opinions from our unique perspective of the world. Not to mention the relentless marketing ads and cell phone alerts that influence us to act on someone else's desire to inform and influence our thinking. Most of our internal perceptions of the outside world have been planted in our minds by outside sources.

Ancient text suggests as a man thinketh in his heart so is he. Our belief about ourselves is the dominant factor in all of our efforts to make concrete changes, to take any positive action, and to incorporate healthier choices of food into our daily routines.

A great question to ask yourself is: "What am I becoming on the road of life that I chose to travel? What results do I observe and is this what I want for my life? Most people's thoughts and beliefs about themselves are destructive, and disempowering, and will ultimately lead them into a place of constant denial, pessimism, fear, shame, and guilt. If you have all of that going on in your life, any kind of positive change will feel like an uphill battle with no end in sight.

Regardless of what our beliefs are, we are being affected by them. Whether they are accurate or not, all you need to do is look around and discern how life looks, and decide if you like what you see. The fact is, it is never what we say that proves our belief; it is always what we do that reveals what we truly believe. The lack of clarity in life leads to indecision, which leads to a false sense of safety. Little do we realize that and not making a choice we are still making a choice.

It has been shown in clinical trials of patients who develop a form of cancer can dramatically impact their recovery based on their mental outlook. Many people who live seemingly healthy and balanced lives show up at the doctor's office for routine checkups and upon hearing of a certain diagnosis, their symptoms now spontaneously arise.

The obvious question is, if there was a cancerous growth in the body why would there be no symptoms until the doctor delivers the news? Your energy can flow where attention is focused. If you believe this is a death sentence then perhaps it is. If you believe this is a lesson in that your new diagnosis serves as a wake-up call to initiate real change and meaningful change that aligns with your predetermined life goals and values this can be your truth. Now I am not suggesting that you ignore the facts of a bad medical report or ignore bad circumstances by pretending they do not exist. No, what I am suggesting is these data points and events in life can serve us in ways that can make us better not bitter. Disease states proliferate in our body in proportion to our belief system surrounding them a cancer could be developing extremely slowly in the body, which could be considered normal, and all of a sudden, it explodes exponentially because someone puts their entire focus on it.

The more we entertain negative thoughts, the more we submit tomorrow's thoughts of the same Association, and the more powerful the emotion behind it becomes, the more deeper rooted those connections become. This is called a neural network of the brain. Research tells us that the human brain is the inspiration behind neural network architecture. Human brain cells, called neurons, form a complex, highly interconnected network and sends electrical signals to each other to help us as humans process information.

The beautiful thing about taking responsibility for the thoughts you are thinking is that no matter how many neuron networks you have formed in a self-destructive manner, you can always pattern in a cut to those connections, and rewire the network receptors by thinking a more positively charged thought.

The brain is constantly reassembling this process in response to the different experiences, emotions, and thoughts we are being exposed to on an immediate basis. If you become self-directed and aware of your thoughts as you are thinking them, then you can alter negative thinking patterns, and replace them with more self-assured, lovely, truth-centered, honest, just, noble, prosperous, virtuous, and exciting thoughts, even when your conscious mind is sleeping. The ancient text describes this as renewing the mind.

Take hold of your mind. Do not fall victim to the whims and shortcomings of others. Understand many of the voices in our head are not our own. They belong to the people who have influenced our life. You may entertain these voices for a time but do not be controlled by them.

Begin reading books or listening to positive audio books and watch videos all that can inspire you and rewire your thinking patterns. Learn new skills that help break old patterns and free our potential. Learning to prepare plant-based meals can be an amazing start on the journey to total health perhaps never realized in your family bloodline. This happened to me. I transformed myself and it started with a thought that led to a decision that led to a plan that led to action steps to include full adoption of a health-centered plant-based eating and a commitment to daily exercise and this new journey is something that I am thoroughly enjoying.

Continually seek out new and healthy ways to consume food as fuel rather than eating food for comfort. This approach to making meals designed to fuel my lifestyle versus food for comfort has changed my life forever. My daily routine is now set in my mind with very little conscious effort.

I prepare most if not all meals from home. I avoid too much packaging in food purchases and I eat mostly organic fruit and vegetables. You might say isn't this expensive? My response was, "I am worth it and I chose to pay now versus later in life when the cost of delayed healthcare can bankrupt even the wealthiest individuals!"

The road to total health has been long, rewarding, and full of exciting turns and twists as I enjoy the new me! I wish this same joyful experience to all who chose to read this writing and apply the principles which when done consistently will assist you in achieving better health, better life choices, and overall a better you!

The transformation starts with a decision to begin a different course in life on a road to health that you must choose for yourself. Remember, there is no substitute for hard work and decision-making aligned with one's values, principles and goals. The steady progressive approach can yield lasting powerful results which include achieving and maintaining an ideal body weight. Better physiological health. Increased energy and clarity of mind to pursue your dreams. You can become a health-conscious physically fit role model to yourself, your family, and your community. The choice is yours and my desire for everyone who reads this writing is to learn that **Health is Wealth** and take the needed action to Own Yours!

THE JOURNEY

Before Plant-Based Decision

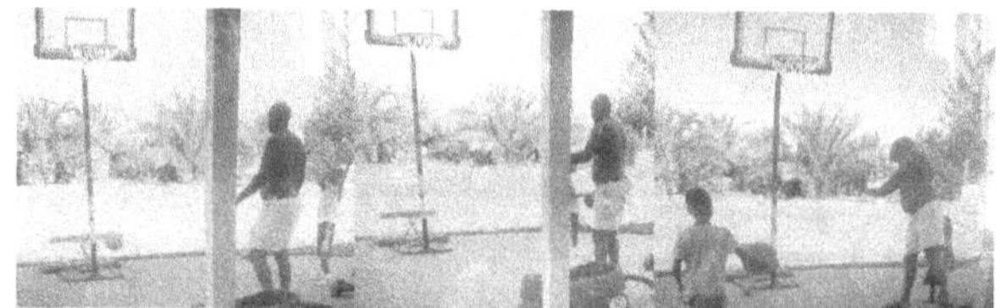

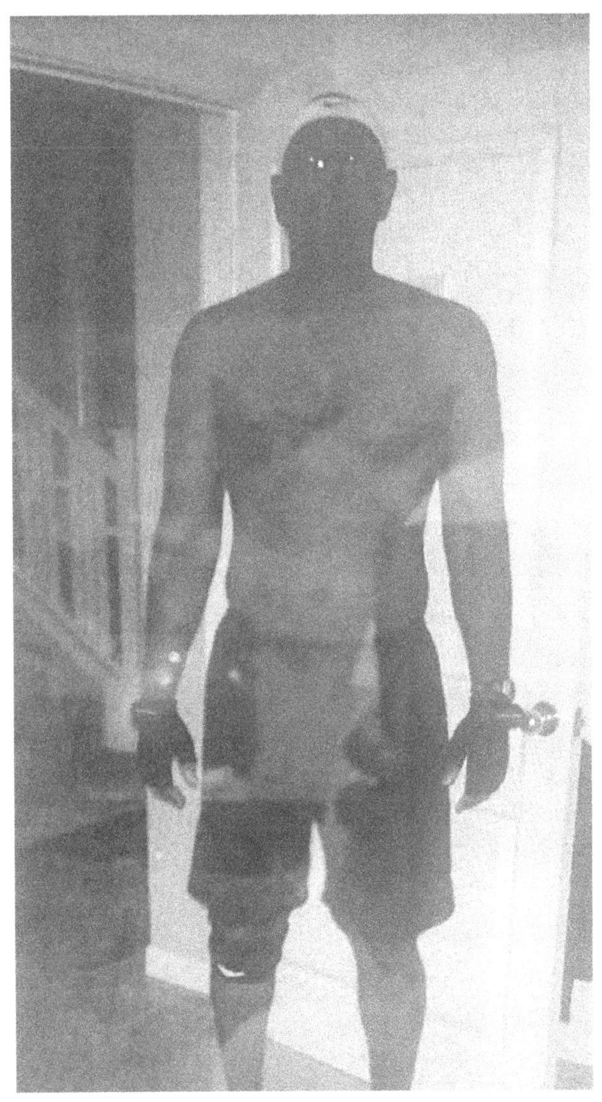

During Transformation Phase 1

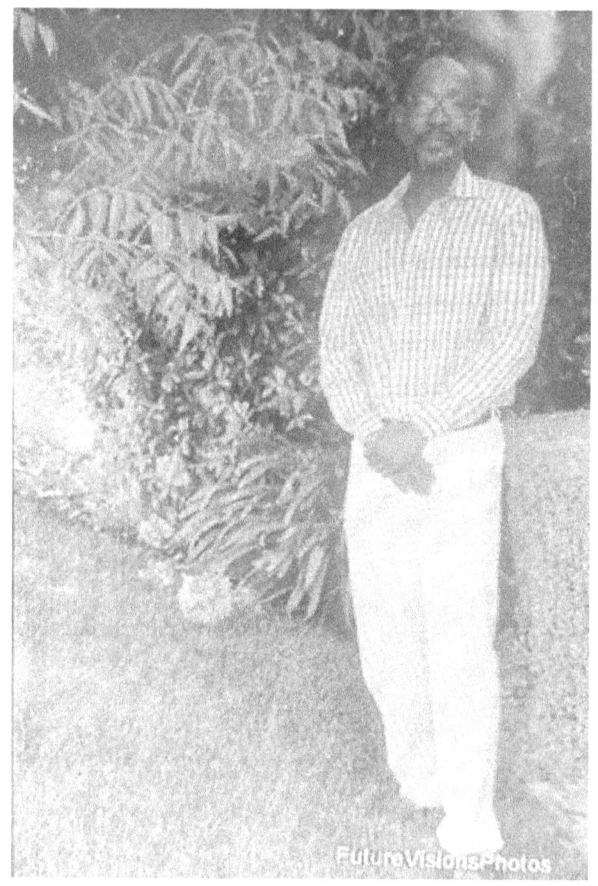
FutureVisionsPhotos

BIBLIOGRAPHY

- **Croft, J. (2023).** *Research Supports Healthy Promise of More Plant-Based Eating*
- **Payer, L. (1992).** *Disease-mongers, how doctors, drug companies, and insurers are making you feel sick: United States.*
- **Sunday Times Times (2016).** *Comfort food according to Collins English Dictionary means soft textures and rich flavors that usually improve with little time and patience.*

ABOUT THE AUTHOR

Carey R Ross Sr.

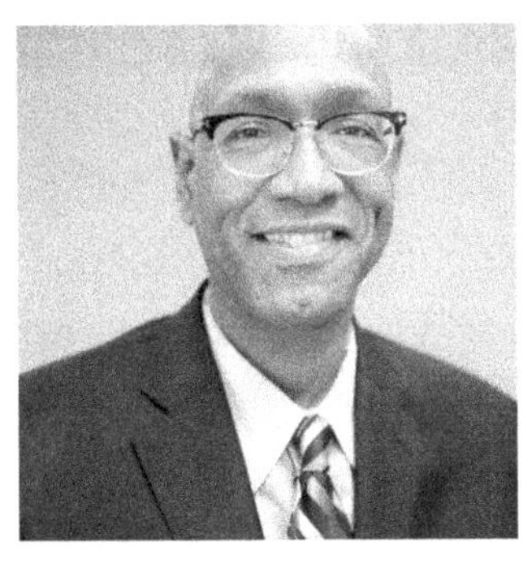 Carey earned his Executive MBA Training Certification from Stanford Graduate School of Business Administration. Carey also earned a Master of Public Administration (MPA) with an emphasis in Healthcare Administration from California State University-Hayward. He also possesses a Bachelor of Science (B.S.) in Business Administration with an emphasis in Business Finance. Carey is also an entrepreneur at heart and is committed to life-long learning.

Carey has served over 35 years in the US Healthcare Industry. Carey started his over 35-year Healthcare career as a contracted nursing professional. Carey has held numerous healthcare delivery leadership roles within the Healthcare Industry.

Carey has a passion for healthcare and as a Senior Regional Leader for Specialty Care, Business Strategy Development, and Technology, Clinical Services, he has led large teams of Operations and Clinical Effectiveness Site

Leaders who have collective accountability for large populations across Northern California.

Carey advances operational execution of prioritized Specialty Services projects that are transforming the Health Care Delivery system to achieve the quadruple aim of improving the health of the population, improving the member experience, reducing cost, and improving the care team wellbeing across select Northern California market areas.

Carey collaborates with Senior Executive Regional Health Care Administrative Leadership for the Continuum of Care, Pharmacy, Clinical Effectiveness, Quality, Care Coordination, Specialty Physician Executives, and other various Regional Leaders including, Health care Finance, Portfolio Management Office, Patient Care Services, and many other Care Delivery teams.

Carey fosters partnerships with other stakeholders including, but not limited to Hospital operations Executives, Marketing & Sales, Health Plan Regulatory Services, Regional Compliance & Public Affairs. He establishes credibility and trust while employing political and business acumen.